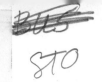

OVERSIZE

OVE

INSTANT
FITNESS

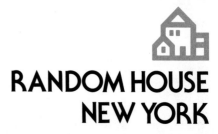

RANDOM HOUSE
NEW YORK

INSTANT FITNESS:

How to Stay Fit and Healthy in Six Minutes a Day

NICHOLAS KOUNOVSKY

Copyright © 1978 by Nicholas Kounovsky
All rights reserved under International and Pan-Ameri-
can Copyright Conventions. Published in the United
States by Random House, Inc., New York, and simultaneously in Canada by Random House of Canada Lim-
ited, Toronto.

Library of Congress Cataloging in Publication Data
Kounovsky, Nicholas Alexis, 1913–
Kounovsky's Instant fitness.
1. Exercise.   2. Physical fitness.   I. Title.
II. Title: Instant fitness.
RA781.K597   613.7'1   77-90303
ISBN 0-394-41316-4

Illustrations by Mickey Surasky

Manufactured in the United States of America
9 8 7 6 5 4 3 2
First Edition

Acknowledgments: I appreciate the patience of my entire family during the writing of this book and the help received from so many of my friends, students and all those who helped experiment with the exercises, pose for photographs and sketches, or demonstrate on TV appearances.

I am grateful to Dr. Vojin N. Smodlaka, sports physician and director of the Department of Rehabilitation Medicine at the Methodist Hospital in Brooklyn, for his comments and advice while discussing problems concerning physical fitness.

Note: Exercises illustrated in strong
yellow are for both men and women, no matter
who appears in the drawing.

Exercises in pale yellow are for women only.

Exercises in black are to be done by
men only.

Contents

Introduction

THE BIRTH OF A METHOD

My interest in physical fitness began as part of a boyhood passion for sports. It was not long after I had been exiled with my parents from Russia to Bulgaria that I became a young "Younak," the Bulgarian term for a boy scout. In Veliko Tyrnovo, where we settled, I spent much time running, climbing and swinging on an exercise device known as "the giant steps" to keep in shape for gymnastics, soccer and track.

I have always been fascinated by motion and energy. After receiving my bachelor's degree from the Sorbonne, I went on to get an engineering degree in aeronautics. However, during those student years in France I never lost interest in athletic and gymnastic training.

As time went on, I began to realize that the movements of the human body were more interesting to me than the dynamics of the airplane. What I really wanted to do was help others achieve the physical fitness that would give them more enjoyment in life. In order to do this, I enrolled in the École Supérieure d'Education Physique in Paris and was later awarded the honorary diploma of the

Ministry of National Education. I was also appointed the chief instructor of the Sokols, the most distinguished organization for physical fitness in Eastern Europe.

Even in 1935 far more was known about machines than about man himself, and, sadly, this is still true today. In reaction to this, I began to put my education in aeronautics to work in a rather revolutionary way by applying the theories of engineering to the human body in motion. In the process I discovered that there is not that much difference between the body and the machine.

During the next five years I had the opportunity to train an unexpected number of fascinating people from all walks of life. Sportspeople and gymnasts, even the sedentary Parisians on whom I practiced my newly born method were able to benefit by and appreciate my techniques.

I particularly remember one man, a well-known horse trainer in Deauville with whom I worked. It was not that he didn't get plenty of exercise working out six horses an hour each a day. But six hours spent gripping the saddle had had a disastrous effect on his thigh muscles. They were strong enough, but so short that off the horse he had to assume the stance of a gorilla. Our sessions together did much for his flexibility—and for his endurance. Thirty years later, when I last saw him, he was still doing handstands and work on the rings at the age of eighty.

And then there was an even more sedentary type—the Parisian businessman who carried out my instant fitness exercises for the chair in the back seat of his Rolls Royce as he was driven from one appointment to the next.

I enjoyed the life in Paris and Deauville, but because I wanted to learn more about what was being done for physical fitness in the "New World," my family and I decided to emigrate to America. I expected to find many new and comprehensive physical fitness programs in the States. Instead, as the physical exams for World War II were soon to show, I discovered that there was as desperate a need for a fitness revolution in America as anywhere else.

New York City was no exception. It has always been a metropolis of abundance and greatness, but it also suffers from the many ills of a big city—with almost as many fads and miracle plans offered as cures for these ills.

With the encouragement of the physical education departments at New York and Columbia Universities, I was confident that I could initiate an effective exercise program in New York and make it successful without using gadgets or gimmicks—only a sound physical and mental approach to fitness.

In spite of a lack of funds—our family capital had dropped from thirty-five to seven dollars in the short period since our arrival—I set out to look for an acceptable space in which to begin my program.

Finally, I found an old apartment that had belonged to the one-time famous actress, Fanny Ward. Covered with inches of dust, it contained nothing but the remnants of a canopy bed and an old silver-fox scarf which I mistook at first for a dead rat. However, it was in an ideal location for my purpose and the owner was willing to rent to me, perhaps because of my enthusiasm and strong belief that I would succeed in my venture.

My wife and I cleaned and painted, and the studio gymnasium was soon ready. All we needed were students. Getting started was a calculated risk. I knew not one person in New York and could barely speak English.

Artists, actors, models and a few doctors soon joined my classes—aware of the importance of their health and looks. In the beginning they were slightly hesitant about coming, but as the days passed and they began to show progress as a result of the training, my program gradually got going as a business. Then a curious incident precipitated my success.

Working on an assignment for *Life* magazine, two of my most faithful students, both models, were asked to stay late and finish the job. During a much-needed rest period the two exhausted young women started a simple relaxation routine they had learned in my classes. The members of the *Life* staff watched with astonishment as the two went through some upside-down exercises. In a few minutes the young women had recharged their batteries through positive relaxation and refreshed by this exercise in "instant fitness," were ready to finish the assignment.

The next day a call came from *Life* inquiring about my program, and a date was set up to take photographs for an article on it. Photographed by my friend Philip Halsman the article, "Engineered Exercise," turned out to be the first of many to appear in national and international publications.

For over three decades several hundred articles have appeared about my work. Since they keep on appearing, it seems safe to assume that I am doing something right.

INSTANT
FITNESS

THE ANATOMY OF INSTANT FITNESS

THE EFFECTS OF NONEXERCISE

The human body is designed to move—and our bodies are not moving enough. Automobiles, elevators and household appliances, even apartment living, are depriving us of adequate physical activity. The result is that our bodies no longer have the ability to go through many of their basic motions.

How many of us can look easily over our shoulders without strain in the muscles of the neck? Or, with any grace or ease, lean down to pick up a dropped subway token? We have become so sedentary that our closely interconnected muscular, nervous, respiratory, circulatory and eliminatory systems are not functioning adequately. And this is precipitating the decline of two of our most treasured assets—youth and fitness.

A PROGRAM OF FITNESS

We can't turn back the clock and banish the automobile along with the apartment dwelling even if we wanted to. However, we can find an antidote to counteract the destructive effects of modern living by following a program of physical fitness based on a well-balanced diet, proper exercise and relaxation.

THE SIXOMETRIC TECHNIQUE

The instant fitness program I have developed concentrates on the six factors that contribute to an excellent body. It is from these six factors that I have coined the term "sixometric" to describe the technique on which my program is based.

These factors are:

Endurance—the resistance of the body to fatigue, which is dependent on the heart and lungs, controlled in the medulla oblongata.

Suppleness—the limberness of the body due to the flexibility of its joints and the elasticity of the muscles, ligaments and tendons.

Equilibrium—the state of body balance and sense of orientation, centered principally in the semicircular canals, directed through the cerebellum and the spinal cord.

Strength—the muscular force of the body, controlled by the cerebro-spinal nervous system.

Speed—the pace of our bodily movements, controlled by the cerebrum.

Skill or coordination—the harmonious function of the physical faculties and the ability of the body to perform movements accurately, controlled in the cerebellum and spinal cord.

Any physical fitness program which neglects or omits any of these six factors is incomplete and insufficient.

REGULARITY AND ENJOYMENT

Physical fitness depends on regular activity—not the kind of spasmodic overexertion which sends many Americans from the tennis court to the intensive care unit. And this activity, to be effective, should be fun, not a chore. Use the instant fitness exercises to put your body in shape to enjoy jogging and other more vigorous forms of exercise in safety.

SIX MINUTES A DAY

Lack of time seems to be the easiest alibi for the lazy nonexerciser. Yet, according to my method, all you have to spend is six minutes a day performing a series of simple movements. Each exercise, which is called a "gymnak," is designed to develop one of the six factors. There are six gymnaks in each set of exercises. By performing at least one set daily, you can be sure that all the important elements in body movement are being developed and improved.

Some of these gymnaks can be done in bed or in the shower; others behind a desk at the office, or in your car. They don't have to be done all at once, but they should be done regularly. A minute here, a minute there during the day, and you'll be surprised how quickly those six minutes add up.

BE YOUR OWN BOSS

In my program the students determine just what and how much they can do. They evaluate their own capacities to perform without strain by giving themselves a series of simple tests. In the same way, they monitor their progress as their physical capacity improves through exercise. They are the ones who decide when they are ready to go on to a more difficult set of gymnaks. Experience has shown us that there is no better incentive to keeping fit than being able to measure one's performance from week to week.

By sticking faithfully to this instant fitness program of only six minutes a day you will soon be aware of your greater stamina and flexibility. Your body will feel younger, more efficient, less tense, and you will have an increased sense of well-being and peace of mind.

WHO SHOULD EXERCISE AND WHY?

The best answer to the question of who should exercise was given to me by the director of the National Institute of Sports in Paris. His response was that "*all* should exercise more as they grow older."

To the question "Why should I exercise?" the answers are many and various. To choose a few at random: to feel well, to look good, to feel more relaxed, to stimulate the circulation, to lose or gain weight . . . But the most important reason is that through exercise we keep our bodies healthy and flexible as we grow older.

EXERCISE AND AGING

As infants we spend most of our waking hours in motion. The physical activity of a youngster is practically nonstop. But as life goes on we tend to reduce these physical activities under the pressure of work and other demands, and soon inactivity becomes a way of life.

Unfortunately, we begin to do this at the very time that we should be increasing our exercise to improve the elimination of waste matters and toxins from our body systems. Effective elimination prevents deposits in the joints and the accompanying stiffening and atrophy that are recognized factors in the aging process. In addition, exercise improves the circulation (which tends to grow sluggish as we grow older), along with our muscular actions and body movements.

Our body is our treasure—something many of us don't realize until the machine begins to fail. To keep it healthy and limber we must give it exercise.

As we learn to speak a language by learning a few words a day, as we give up smoking by eliminating one more cigarette a day, or lose unwanted weight by cutting out a few ounces of food a day, so can we, by exercising a few minutes a day, keep our bodies fit. It is hard to believe how so little effort can achieve so much.

IS IT EVER TOO LATE?

Many students who come to the studio on their first visit ask anxiously "Is it too late for me to start? Can I repair the damage caused by lack of exercise?" The answer is *no* to the first and *yes* to the second question. As long as we have medical approval it is never too late (or too soon!) to start a physical fitness program.

At one of his last lectures Dr. Paul Dudley White, a man who gave so much to the cause of physical fitness, said "It is fascinating to know that one can grow healthier as one grows older. Not necessarily the reverse."

I have had students over eighty and vanity being what it is, I wouldn't be surprised if some were even older. The youngest was three and a half, the son of the Aga Khan, who used to enjoy coming to watch his child perform in my studios in Deauville and in Paris, but refused to become a convert to exercise himself.

BEFORE YOU BEGIN

Most of us take good care of our cars—we have to. Every year a sticker is required, confirming that the car has been checked, adjusted and approved, thus ensuring that it will stay in good shape, be safer and last longer.

CHECK OUT YOUR BODY MACHINE

In the same way we should check our body machine before embarking on an instant fitness program. The machine's engine (the cardiovascular system), its mechanical faculties (muscles and joints), its electrical system (nerves), should all be checked against the medical standards for physical fitness, without forgetting to check the fuel and lubrication (nutrition).

So be sure to see your doctor for a check-up before you begin the instant fitness program. This is the golden rule of any physical fitness routine.

PROCEED WITH CAUTION

Even after you have received a clean bill of health from your doctor, proceed as if you were a convalescent, especially if you have been inactive for a long time, or if you are a beginner at exercising. This may sound overcautious, but unmoderated physical effort often leads to physical setbacks. And remember, you have only one body.

4 | ENERGIZING YOUR EXERCISE

We know that all physical activity, such as walking, climbing, jumping, throwing, carrying, running, lifting, pushing, pulling, bending, twisting, stretching and even blinking an eyelid, requires energy. The fact is, you can consume fifty calories an hour just by standing still.

But to expend energy we must first have it. To have it, we need food with proper nutrients.

CHOOSING YOUR DIET

Choosing a sensible, nutritious diet tailored to our individual needs can be quite a problem. One of the difficulties is the number of popular diets that appear every so often and sweep the country. Low fat, high protein, low cholesterol, vegetarian, high fiber, semifasting—the array is bewildering. And yet not one of these diets is able to give us a clear formula for what is best for us personally.

Even in the world of medical research there are continuing controversies and differences of opinion about diet. Some reports show that we consume excessive amounts of meat but not enough of the other necessary foods; others indicate that it is not so much what we eat as how we assimilate it.

SEE YOUR DOCTOR

Since a thorough discussion of diet is beyond the scope of this book, my advice is to discuss the subject with your doctor when you have your medical checkup before beginning the instant fitness program. It is important to make sure that you are getting all the nutrients your body needs. In our affluent society the danger is not so much *under*nourishment as it is *over*nourishment or *mal*nourishment.

REFUELING

Assuming, then, that you are well nourished, the important factor is the quantity of food consumed. This quantity should be balanced with the amount of energy your body requires.

The formula will always remain the same: intake should equal expenditure to maintain the status quo. Whether you gain or lose weight will be determined by the difference in intake over expenditure (energy spent), and expenditure over intake.

A vivid example of energy input and output is a man who gained twelve pounds in one year simply because he had received a promotion which entitled him to park his car in the executive parking lot, some five hundred feet closer to the office than the place where he used to leave it.

A WORD TO DIETERS

To those of you who wish to lose weight, don't begin to diet before you start on your instant fitness program. Weight loss through diet alone causes loss of fitness, and you will need to compensate for that by starting on your fitness exercises *before,* not after you begin to cut down on your food intake.

HOW MUCH EXERCISE?

The suggested daily six-minute exercise period is the minimum time for achieving fitness. You may, of course, add as many six-minute periods as you wish, especially if your aim is to lose weight. But again, remember not to overdo it. Be aware of your body and watch for signs of fatigue.

REST AND RECUPERATION

Almost as important as sound nutrition is rest. Our bodies need just enough rest for recuperation—that sense of satisfaction that we feel after a good night's sleep or even a brief rest during the day.

Another point to remember is that some of us are night people, others are up and ready to go early in the morning. Accept your inner clock, but be sure to get the amount of rest that is right for you.

It's worth mentioning, too, that there is such a thing as "negative rest"—the kind that brings on a sense of listlessness and can weaken and atrophy the body systems. How much rest you actually need can easily be measured by your general feeling of vigor and well-being.

5 RELAX AND TRY

Before you take the evaluation tests it is important to realize that you may not have tried some of the movements for weeks, months, years —or possibly never.

TAKE IT EASY

It is probable that your muscles, tendons and ligaments have not been stretched sufficiently, so in your self-evaluation exercises proceed with caution. Don't force it. Stop at the point just approaching that feeling of having to force. Any overstretch, overwork or overstrain will only delay your progress or, worse still, could make you decide to give up exercising. The point of the evaluation tests is to find out how much you can do without strain, what you cannot do, and what you could do better.

BEGIN CAUTIOUSLY

Chronological age is a factor to consider. As an older beginner, you can't expect to do as well on the evaluation tests as a younger person whose body has not had as much time to stiffen. But young or old, if your body is not trained to a regular fitness program you would be wise to consider yourself a convalescent or even an invalid as you begin the exercises.

Quite often at a party or other friendly gathering the topic of conversation turns to fitness. Invariably, after a minute or two of discussion the entire assembly is in action trying to execute a knee bend, or touch the floor with the palms of the hands, etc. Cries of "I used to be able to do it" or "I never *could* do that" fill the crowded room. The result is that the next day most of those people remember their attempts with a sore thigh, a tender abdomen, or a pulled shoulder.

Every summer in my gymnastic organization we close down our activities for a few months. At the beginning of the fall session I always remind my friends that in spite of all the tennis, swimming and other outdoor sports most of them participated in over the summer, it is possible that they did not bend or stretch as much as they do in our program, and so they should begin cautiously.

An I-know-better smile usually appears on their faces—until the moment when we execute a deep knee bend and a barrage of cracks and pops is heard. Then the smiles disappear and everyone is convinced of the truth of my warning.

THE SIXOMETRIC TECHNIQUE

To determine your state of fitness I have come up with some simple and practical gymnaks designed to show you how possible it is for you to perform certain movements.

SPOTTING YOUR WEAKNESSES

Remember that the results of these self-evaluation exercises only indicate what you are capable of doing at the time you try them. Use the results to plot a course to increase your competence in all six factors: Endurance, Suppleness, Equilibrium, Strength and Speed, and aim for their perfect control through Coordination.

In spotting your weaknesses and in planning for their improvement, don't jump to the conclusion that instant fitness will do the trick immediately. What it can do is set you instantly on the right track by giving you the choice and direction through which to achieve complete fitness.

Take your time and carefully analyze each gymnak. Gradually you will learn the best way to perform it and to improve the factor involved.

FINDING YOUR OWN RHYTHM

To do all the exercises in the same rhythm is a mistake, and can even be harmful. Also, the tedium that results is a drawback to enjoyment.

The great majority of physical education instructors fail to understand that each student must follow his or her own rhythm, amount and kind of exercise rather than conform to what suits the instructor's abilities and habits.

So be your own instructor and stick to a procedure that suits your needs best and fulfills the main purpose of your program—to find out what your body can and cannot do.

7

TEST YOUR OWN FITNESS

HOW TO PROCEED

Without straining, perform each of the following tests for the six factors in body excellence. Then analyze what motions you can or cannot perform. Make a notation after each gymnak so that when you are through you can see at a glance which are your areas of weakness and strength. Don't worry if at first you can't do them all. Even if you do them incompletely you will be well on your way to instant fitness.

To check your endurance

The most important factor in general fitness is endurance, or resistance to fatigue, which is determined by your cardiovascular system, your heart, lungs and blood circulation. It can be evaluated by measuring your thoracic capacity (lungs), your heartbeat (pulse) and your heart response to exercise.

To enjoy the instant fitness program without fatigue you must be in reasonably good condition. It also helps to have healthy lungs and a strong heart.

To check your breathing

Before evaluating your lung capacity, check your breathing
habits:

• Do you breathe correctly when
you exercise, inhaling through the
nostrils, exhaling through the
mouth?

• Do you hold your breath when
you should not?

• Do you breathe deeply enough
when needed?

Ask yourself:

• Do I get enough fresh air?

• Do I get enough physical work
for my heart and lungs?

Now go ahead with the first test.

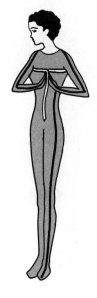

To check your lung capacity

1. Take a deep breath and hold it.
Then, with a tape, measure the circumference of your chest at the
level of the breast bone. Mark the
measurement down. Exhale as
much air as possible and measure
your chest circumference again.
Compare the two measurements
and note the difference. It should
be approximately two-and-a-half
inches for women and three-and-a-
half inches for men. The greater
the difference, the better your lung
capacity.

2. The Apnea Test: Take a deep
breath and hold it for as long as
possible. Note the time. (The average is fifty-five seconds.)

Then, exhale and don't take an-

other breath for as long as you
can. Note the time. (The average is
fifteen seconds.)

To check your heart activity
The activity of the heart is measured by the number of beats a
minute, or pulse rate. A well-
trained heart with strong muscles
pumps blood steadily and effi-
ciently. Therefore, it is advisable to
train your heart to be efficient and
strong through exercise. Normally,
the pulse averages 70–75 beats per
minute, the closer to 70 the better.
1. To check the *pace of your
heart beat:*

Take your pulse at rest. On the
inside of your left wrist locate the
artery, and delicately cover it with
the tips of the first three fingers of
your right hand. Let your right
thumb rest gently against the outside
of your wrist. Now count your beats.

You can take your pulse for fifteen seconds and multiply the
number of beats by four, or for
thirty seconds and multiply by two.
For the most accurate count take
your pulse for a full sixty seconds.

Normally, the pulse varies, de-
pending upon your position (if
you're lying, sitting or standing),
your food consumption (if you've
just eaten or had a cup of coffee),
and your general condition (if
you've just rested, or had a rough
day or night).

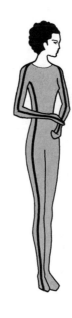

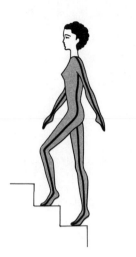

2. To check your *heart response:*
Take your pulse and make a note of it. According to your ability, walk up an average of two flights of stairs, two steps per second. Retake your pulse when you reach the top. Keep taking it every minute, and note when the heart rate returns to normal.

> One minute or less—excellent
> Two minutes—good
> Three minutes—average
> Four minutes—fair
> Five minutes or over—poor

Through the weeks of training, your fitness will improve, your heart rate will slow down at rest and return faster to normal after all of the above tests.

3. The Orange Test.
Place a twenty-inch high stepstool or a chair close to a wall or other support. Try to step on and off the stool twelve times in thirty seconds.
Take your pulse sixty seconds after stopping.
If the heartbeat is below one hundred you are in good shape.

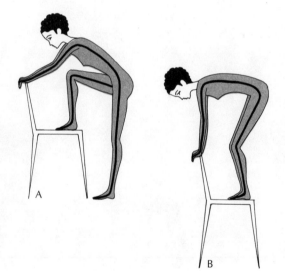

To check your suppleness

In order to bend easily and move freely all your joints and articulations should be given a chance to move and remain limber. To check your suppleness or flexibility, evaluate the major angular motions in the following gymnaks.

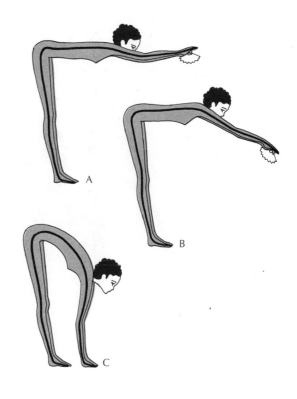

For your shoulders and posture

From a standing position, if possible facing a mirror, bend your body forward at the hips. Keep your back straight and parallel to the floor, your head up, on a line with your back.

Holding a yardstick or a broomstick at shoulder level, try to extend your arms straight forward and up, raising the ruler or broomstick to the level of your eyes without lowering it.

If the stick is above your eyes—
very good
Close to eye level—fair
Below eye level—poor

For your forward spine and hip suppleness

From standing position, feet together—comfortably, without bending your knees or straining—bend your torso forward and try to reach the floor with your hands.

Touching the floor palms down
—very good
Just touching the floor with fingertips—fair
Not touching the floor—poor

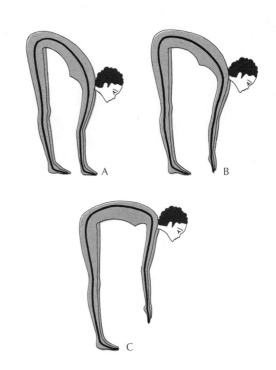

For your hip and leg flexibility.

Stand, left hand on support, right arm stretched forward at eye level. Lifting your right leg, try to touch your fingers with your toes. Repeat on left side.

Touching with ease—very good
If toes are five to ten inches
below your hand—fair
More than ten inches—poor

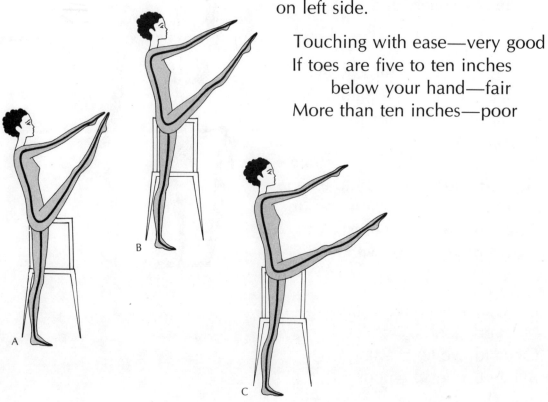

For your backward spine and leg suppleness

Lying flat in a prone position, bend your knees, reach back and try to grasp your ankles with your hands. Proceed gently and don't force it. If you're not that supple, don't be discouraged.

Holding ankles—very good
Just touching ankles—fair
Not getting near ankles—poor

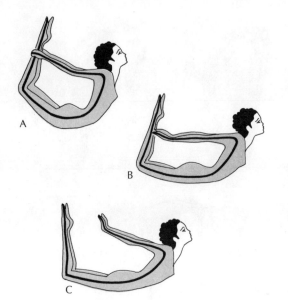

To check your equilibrium

For your balance and stability
With eyes closed, arms stretched out at the sides, standing on one foot, the other knee bent and up, try to remain in balance without shifting or shuffling your supporting foot. Try the same for the other leg and note the times.

For ten seconds or over
—very good
Six to ten seconds—fair
Five seconds or less—poor

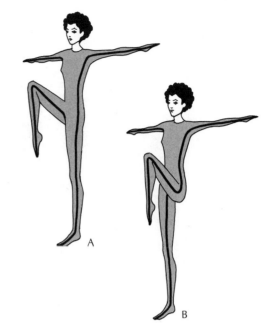

Balance in motion (static position)
Standing on one foot, try the three poses illustrated—controlling the balance for at least three seconds in each pose, without shuffling your supporting foot.

All three poses—very good
Two poses—fair
One or none—poor

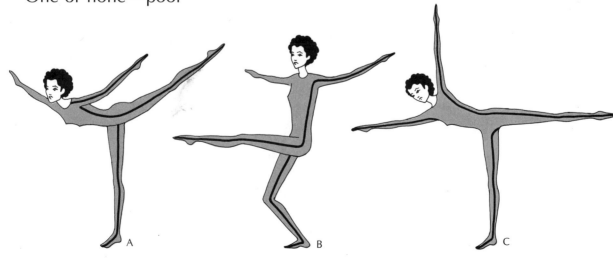

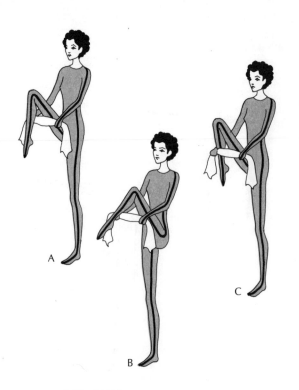

Balance in motion with orientation

Stand and hold a towel taut in front of you at the level of your hips. Maintaining your balance, slowly pass one foot inside and over the towel, then return to the original position. Repeat same with the other leg.

> Both legs passed with ease —very good
> Only one leg—fair
> Bending but not passing—poor

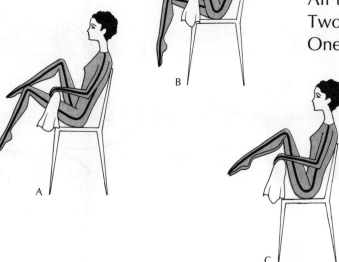

Sitting in balance

Sit on the edge of a chair, holding a towel taut in front of you. Balancing on your hips, feet off the floor, try to pass one leg after the other over the towel. Now try to pass both legs over the towel simultaneously.

> All three tests—very good
> Two of the three—fair
> One or none—poor

To check your strength

To handle physical effort without stress or strain, all your muscles, the providers of motion, must be at their maximum efficiency. Your physical strength and power is in direct relation to your muscular development.

To evaluate the strength of your wrists (handgrip) and arms
Try to hang from a rope or from the top of an open door; women use both hands, men use one. If you are using the door, open it all the way and place a wedge under the bottom to lock it and prevent pull on the hinges. Place a towel on the top of the door to ease the strain on your hands.

Hanging for more than fifteen
seconds—very good
Five to fifteen—fair
Less than five—poor

In addition, men should try to chin-up with both arms.

More than ten chin-ups
—very good
Five to ten—fair
Less than five—poor

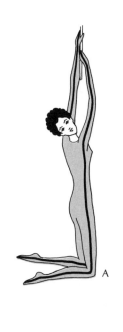

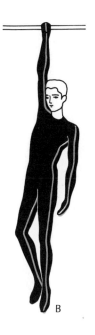

To evaluate pushing power

FOR WOMEN—in a prone position, on one knee and one foot, the other leg extended, hands flat on the floor with your arms bent and your chin touching the floor, push simultaneously with your hands and foot, lifting your body three times from the floor. Repeat with the other leg.

Simultaneous lift—very good
Alternating lift (two steps)—fair
Only arms or leg—poor

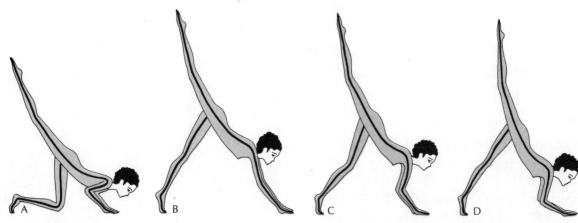

FOR MEN—heels against the wall or any stopper (such as a couch, closed door or a bed), hands on the floor at a specific distance (the distance from the wall to the fingertips should be half your height), arms bent, the top of the head on the floor or on a towel, try to perform three push-ups, keeping your legs straight.

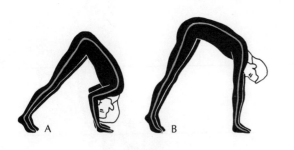
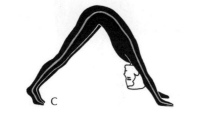

At indicated distance
    —very good
Three-quarters of your height
    —fair
Farther out—poor

To evaluate abdominal strength

1. From a lying position on your back, arms overhead, swing your arms forward and try to sit up. If successful:

2. Try to simultaneously raise one leg and reach the toes with the opposite hand. If successful:

3. Place your hands behind your neck and try simultaneously to sit up, raise your bent knees and reach them with your elbows.

For test 3—very good
For test 2—fair
For test 1 only—poor

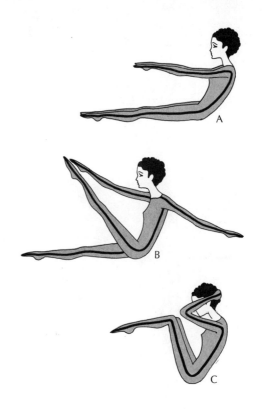

To evaluate the strength of your legs

1. Holding on to the back of a chair or to a doorknob, slowly try to do two or three knee bends.

2. Without holding on, try a full knee bend.

3. If you feel up to it, try a one-knee bend.

For test 3—very good
For test 2—fair
For test 1 only—poor

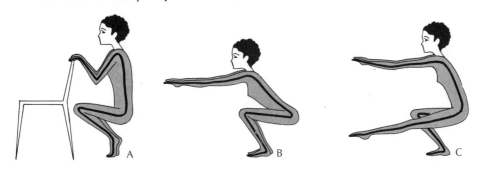

To check your speed

To react swiftly, to dodge a reckless driver and avert an accident, our initial and maximum speeds must be at their peak.

Today everything moves faster. Not just to keep up with the times, but perhaps for our very survival, we must adjust our speed factor accordingly.

To evaluate your initial speed

Put three coins on the top surface of your forearm. Cast them up, and as rapidly as possible try to catch them one after the other before they drop.

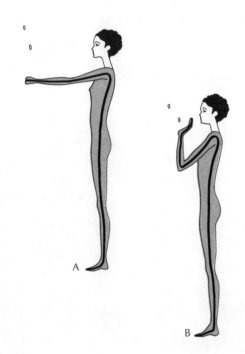

> If you catch all three
> —very good
> If you catch two—fair
> If you catch one—poor

To evaluate your maximum speed

Pin a sheet of paper on the wall about twelve inches above your head level. Standing sideways to the wall, legs apart, try to touch—as fast as possible—first the paper, then the outside foot. Keep touching for ten seconds, counting the move from paper to foot to paper as one movement.

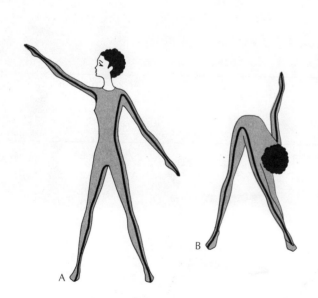

> More than ten times in
> ten seconds—very good
> From six to ten—fair
> Five or less—poor

To check your skill or coordination

This is obviously the most complex factor to evaluate as there are so many different physical skills to test. Nevertheless, a few simple exercises will give a general evaluation of how well coordinated you are.

1. Lunge forward several times and come back, each time changing leg and raising the opposite arm.

First attempt—good
Second attempt—fair
Third attempt—poor

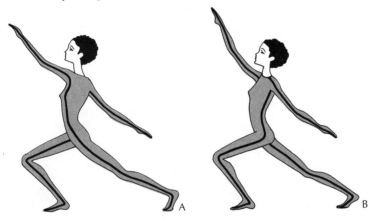

2. Lying in a prone position, arms and legs stretched out and up, slowly bend one arm, pushing the elbow back as far as it will go, and simultaneously bend the opposite leg. Alternate arms and legs.

First attempt—good
Second attempt—fair
Third attempt—poor

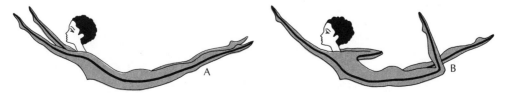

3. From a standing position, perform the movements of the breast stroke. Carefully study the sequence.

A. Stretch your arms above your head, back of the hands together, palms out.

B. Stretch arms sideways at a level with the shoulders.

C. Bend your knees in the crouch position, simultaneously bring your palms together at a level with your breastbone, elbows out.

D. Jump, legs wide apart, arms extended above the head, palms together.

Perform all four portions in a continuous manner.

First attempt—good
Second attempt—fair
Third attempt—poor

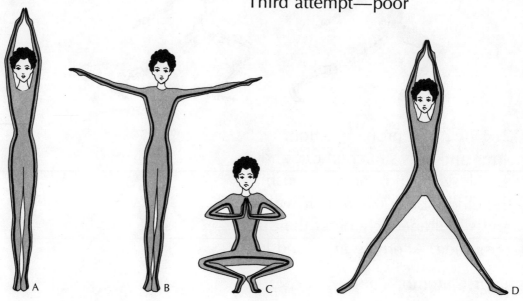

8

HOW TO EXERCISE

HAVE A PLAN OF ACTION

After evaluating your state of fitness, determine your plan of action and proceed with it regularly.

Exercise can be harmful or, at the very least, useless if you do not know how to do it correctly. A wrongly executed or excessive work-out may lead to fatigue and stress (today's enemy) or even to the gradual acceleration of the aging process by causing deterioration in the body tissues.

Too many strength exercises, especially for women, may develop unsightly bulging muscles and decrease suppleness and speed.

Too many flexibility exercises can overstretch the ligaments and tendons, weakening the joints and general bodily strength.

AVOIDING STRAIN

Overdoing may jeopardize our health. This is why jogging, active or violent sports, and "pushed" calisthenics should be preceded by a comprehensive "get ready" fitness program like the one described in this book.

It is unwise to suddenly run or jump or jog for an hour before developing and firming a reasonably strong abdominal girdle and, what is even more important, training the heart to endure stress—even of the lighter kind.

WHAT, HOW AND HOW MUCH

What, how and how much are the keys to sensible exercise. Each movement should be done with a purpose: for strength, suppleness, endurance, etc. That purpose determines how the movement is carried out—its rhythm, intensity, continuity, duration and its amplitude of motion and position.

DON'T BE SLOPPY

All exercises should be performed as precisely and attractively as possible. Don't be sloppy. Keep your head up, knees straight, your toes pointed and hands and fingers aligned, unless the directions indicate otherwise. Your head should follow the line of the spine—forward when the spine is rounded, backward when it is arched.

The beauty in exercising is the ease of performance and the coordination of all the body movements during a particular gymnak. Breathing, posture, gait, facial expression, even the hands and feet can be expressive in any given exercise.

WORKING UP

It is very important for the body to perform every motion at least six times to give it a fair chance for fitness. With that aim in mind begin by trying each exercise once, gradually working up from one to six times.

If an exercise becomes too easy, shift to a more challenging one. Or increase the intensity of the exercise—sometimes the number of times you do it, sometimes the rhythm, sometimes deliberately holding difficult positions, sometimes varying the rest periods.

Proportion your activity to your capacity. If you can't do a certain gymnak at first, forget about it until your fitness improves. Or, if you aren't up to completing a gymnak, do part of it. For example, take the gymnak for suppleness on p. 23. If at first you can't touch the floor with palms down, bring your hands down as far as they *will* go. Even if it is only an inch or two below your kneecaps, leave it at that for the time being. As your flexibility improves you will be able to go further and eventually you will be able to complete the gymnak by touching the floor with your palms or at least with your fingertips.

EXERCISE SHOULD BE FUN

To be effective, the fitness session or workout should not be a chore. There should be no hurry, stress or strain. It should last just long enough to make you feel good and stimulated, but relaxed—with the incentive to continue regularly. Never push to the point of exhaustion. Nothing destroys incentive as much as fatigue.

1998382

9 BREATHING

All of us breathe all the time—and most of us assume that we are doing it correctly. Alas, this is not always true.

To successfully learn a stroke in tennis or a step in dancing, we have to concentrate, study and sometimes practice a long time. The same is true of breathing. And no wonder. There are as many as seventeen breathing muscles (muscles of respiration) that come into play as we breathe. To pay close attention and get these muscles to work fully and harmoniously is not an easy task, but it is essential to any form of exercise. Nevertheless, we often fail to concentrate on our breathing.

BREATHING DURING EXERCISE

To help our bodies function at their best while exercising, breathing should be carried out by inhaling through the nose—as when smelling a flower, and then exhaling through the mouth—as when blowing out a candle. Yet it is not uncommon to see a ballet dancer backstage panting like a dog, mouth wide open, inhaling into her lungs all the dust and impurities from the wings, instead of first filtering the air through her nostrils. (In swimming, inhaling should be done with your mouth and exhaling through nose and mouth, or mouth alone.)

RHYTHM

The rhythm of breathing should correspond to, or at least come close to matching the degree to which the body demands oxygen. The greater the need, the faster or deeper the breathing. However, it is useless to breathe rapidly when the body doesn't require a great deal of oxygen. It will only tire you unnecessarily and interfere with your progress.

Synchronize the rhythm of breathing with the intensity of your effort. When the chest is involved, try to exhale at the moment that the chest wall is compressed, and inhale when the chest is expanded, making a bellowslike motion.

In protracted and continuous physical effort the rhythm of breathing should be adapted to match the effort that is being expended.

OUT OF BREATH

After vigorous activity, when we seem to be out of breath and stop for a lungful of fresh air, it is better to exhale deeply to rid the lungs of as much of the impure air (carbon dioxide) as possible before taking a deep breath.

10

SIXOMETRIC GUIDANCE

Now that your capacity for physical fitness has been evaluated and established, let's talk about the necessity for a regular and methodical fitness program.

Every day, just as you eat, sleep, wash and brush your teeth, you must exercise all the fitness factors if:

• you don't want to tire easily, get out of breath and puff after a simple effort.

• you don't want to be stiff and inflexible, have difficulty getting into a taxi, or leaning down to put on your shoes.

• you don't want to lose your balance on a stool putting up curtains, or stepping onto an escalator while you're out shopping.

• you don't want to be too weak to open a jammed door or a tightly capped jar, lift a garbage can or carry your own suitcase.

• you don't want to be slow, sluggish and unable to cope with fast-moving traffic and the tempo of city life.

• you don't want to be awkward, clumsy, inefficient and unable to perform all body movements harmoniously.

The evaluation tests will pinpoint your weaknesses and help you choose the kind of exercises you need. Your needs will determine the procedure; the Sixometric techniques will do the rest.

WORKING ON YOUR WEAKNESSES

According to your findings, proceed gymnak by gymnak to work on your weak points.

When exercising for *endurance* pay special attention to your breathing. With each exercise make sure that you are carrying out a complete expiration and full inspiration that extends from the thoracic to the diaphragmatic and to the abdominal regions, limbering the shoulder girdle, the ribs and the spine.

In addition to your sets, do some brisk walking. Go out of your way to climb a flight of stairs or two, and once your instant fitness program is under way, include in your leisure time some kind of active sport. In a short while you will notice that a marvelous change has taken place in your entire body: your heart and lungs will be more active and therefore healthier and stronger, and your circulation will begin to respond to your increased capacity for fresh air.

When exercising for *suppleness* make sure that all movements are performed to the fullest extent. Each time you attempt to stretch, bend or twist, be sure that each movement is a *complete* one. At the same time, check to make certain that all opposing muscles are relaxed.

By accentuating, little by little, all your movements you will begin to feel the rewarding effects of a supple body.

When exercising for equilibrium, pay special attention to your center of gravity, the crucial point in maintaining perfect balance in either a static or moving position. Practice with your eyes open and then closed, guiding all changes in position according to your center of gravity.

When exercising for *strength,* make sure that you are completely contracting and relaxing each muscle involved. Be aware of this whenever you are running, climbing, jumping, throwing, carrying, pushing, lifting and pulling, or just walking.

When exercising for *speed,* concentrate on rapid movements in every region of the body. Separate each part and increase its speed. Then combine two parts—for instance, the arms and the legs—working up to maximum speed. Each time you exercise, especially in your specific speed gymnaks, accelerate your tempo.

When exercising for *skill and coordination,* pay attention to each factor separately, then combine them in sequences; for instance, speed with endurance, or suppleness with coordination, using only the necessary muscles involved in each factor. Perfect your movements by trying as many different exercises as possible.

Supplement the exercises with games, sports and other activities that require precision. Add some simple routines of your own, such as putting on your stockings or lacing your shoes while balancing on one leg. You might also try doing these with your eyes shut. Or while you are walking on the street make believe you are traversing an imaginary beam or tightrope.

RHYTHM AND INTENSITY

The rhythm and intensity with which an exercise is done has an important effect on its value. How you decide to do a certain exercise depends, first, on how fit you are and second, on what you want from it: speed, endurance, suppleness, etc. Each factor requires a different rhythm, and sometimes the chosen rhythm may take a little time to attain. As a beginner, even if you are working for speed, begin slowly and work up.

As for intensity, every exercise can be done intensively or relaxedly, using a minimum or maximum of effort. Many other factors can change the intensity of an exercise: the position in which it is done, the resistance involved, the leverage, etc.

QUANTITY

Each set of gymnaks represents a small entity, in which there are six exercises with specific objectives for each factor. One set of these each day will help keep "unfitness" away, several sets will put you into even better shape. Just as in tennis where one set is helpful, several sets will be even more beneficial, provided you don't push to the point of exhaustion.

For your fitness program select your minimum set of gymnaks for the day. To speed up the improvement of the factors that need working on, gradually add a few more. The more difficult exercises should not be attempted until you have worked up to them.

NUMBER OF REPETITIONS

The number of times an exercise is performed depends on your honesty about what you need and/or your capacity. Ideally, each exercise in each set should be done six times, but as a beginner use your judgment about how much of a particular exercise you have the capacity for. If you are beginning to feel a strain, stop.

SPACING

Once the rhythm, intensity and quantity of an exercise is established, you must decide how to space them. The interval of rest between each exercise, and between two different exercises, can affect the restoration of your normal heart beat and replenish oxygen in the lungs. So take time to rest.

RX FOR OVERSTRAIN

If after a few days of exercises you suddenly feel slightly stiff and perhaps a little sore, in spite of the precautions you have taken to avoid overdoing, the chances are that you have overworked or overstretched a bit. The soreness and stiffness should disappear with some light exercises of the muscles involved to bring the flow of blood back to the affected areas.

Let us say your shoulder is a little stiff and sore. To avoid further stress stop doing any of the gymnaks that involve the shoulder girdle. Instead, begin daily to gently rotate your shoulders. Not in wide circles, but just enough to get the circulation going where the muscles may have been slightly overstretched. Continue to do this until the stiffness is gone and you can resume your regular exercises without strain or discomfort.

Treat an elbow, knee, or any other part suffering from overexercising, in the same way.

11

THE GYMNAKS

In my boy-scout days the rule for rising in the morning was "get up like a jumping jack." However, experience has taught me that a reasonable transition from immobility to activity is the best way to avoid surprises. After a night's sleep all the body systems function at a slow pace and the circulation is idling—less than a quarter of our blood vessels are at work. So it helps if the blood circulation has a chance to adjust from a lying to a standing position.

For this reason the first set of gymnaks is designed to get you off to a good start with some mild activity while you are still in bed.

Each gymnak will take you from three to five seconds. Repeated six times, it should take from eighteen to thirty seconds. Thus, a set of gymnaks will amount to approximately three minutes a set.

By performing one more set during the day—at your desk, waiting in the car, at home with a towel or a broom—you can increase your activity time to six minutes.

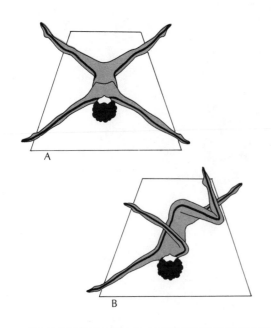

INSTANT FITNESS ON THE BED

1. For your endurance: Lying on your back, arms and legs outstretched, inhale. Slowly move your right arm to the left across your chest. Simultaneously bend your left knee and bring it to the right across your body. Exhale. Alternate arms and legs.

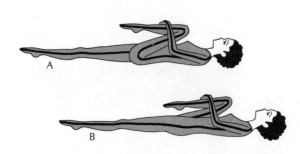

2. For your suppleness: Lie flat on your back, legs together and your body loose and relaxed. Inhale deeply. Then slowly bend your left knee, grasp and hug it with both hands, gently pulling it toward your body as you exhale. Release your leg and come back to the relaxed position. Inhale and repeat with the right leg.

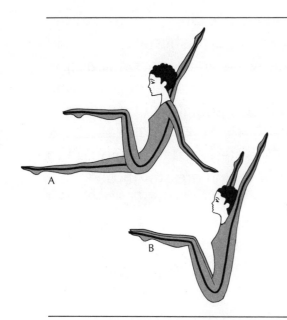

3. For your equilibrium: Sitting on the bed, arms back, leaning on your outstretched hands, slowly bend one knee and raise one arm. Then, lift both feet off the bed, raise both arms and try to balance on your hips from ten to thirty seconds. Return slowly to a sitting position and repeat. Breathe deeply and slowly.

4. For your strength: Lie in bed with hands clasped behind your neck, knees bent, feet apart. Slowly; pressing with your feet, raise your hips while gently arching your back. Inhale going up, exhale coming down.

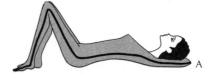

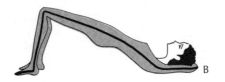

5. For your speed: Leaning back on your elbows, bending the knees with feet off the bed, imitate the motion of bicycle riding. Breathe deeply. Repeat several times, accelerating the tempo to improve leg velocity.

6. For your coordination: Arms back, leaning on your hands, inhale deeply. Simultaneously place your right hand on the back of your head and bend your left knee. Now try to reach your left knee with your right elbow or, if you are very good, with your shoulder. Exhale. Come back to the original position. Inhale and repeat on the opposite side.

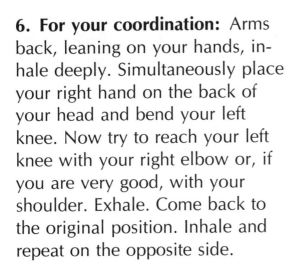

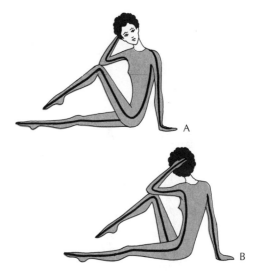

INSTANT FITNESS IN THE SHOWER

During the night, beside resting, the body continues its elimination through the pores. In the morning, mild exercises in the shower will increase the circulation and cleanse and open the pores. (Be sure you have a nonslip floor surface in the shower or a rubber mat to stand on.)

If you exercise while the shower is running, remember to change your method of breathing. Instead of inhaling through your nose, breathe with your mouth, as in swimming.

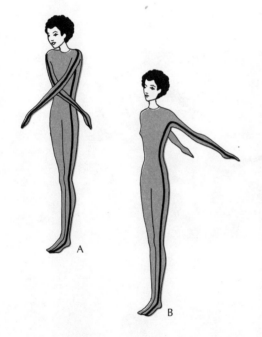

7. For your endurance: In standing position, take a deep breath. Slowly bring your arms and shoulders forward, squeezing your chest and exhaling completely. Slowly move your arms and shoulders back and inhale. Repeat the exercise.

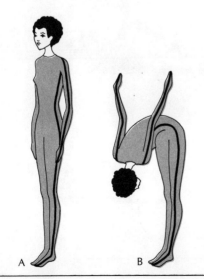

8. For your suppleness: From a standing position, take a deep breath, then slowly bend your body forward, moving your arms back and up as you exhale completely. Slowly straighten up. Inhale and repeat the exercise.

9. For your equilibrium: From a standing position, hands on hips, bend your right knee, and slowly raise your right foot behind you. Try to balance for ten seconds and, if possible, close your eyes. Do the same with the left foot. Breathe slowly and deeply.

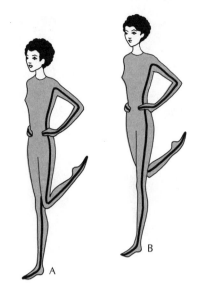

10. For your strength: Standing in a slightly crouched position, hands on knees, slowly bend and then extend your legs, gently pressing with your hands. Breathe regularly, exhaling when bent, inhaling when extended.

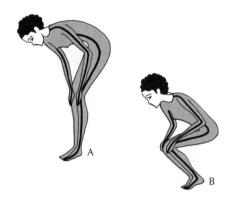

11. For your speed: In standing position, bend one arm after the other at the elbow, accelerating the tempo. Breathe with every two to six motions of the arms.

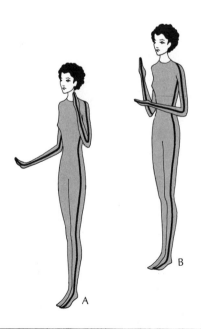

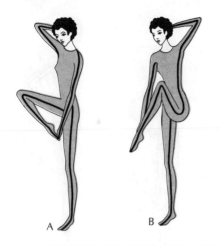

12. For your coordination: Left hand behind your neck, inhale deeply, then slowly bend your left knee and raise it high, trying to reach your toes with your right hand as you gently twist your body. Exhale as you straighten up. Change arm and repeat with the other leg.

INSTANT FITNESS WITH A TOWEL

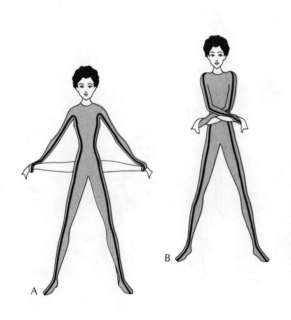

A towel is an excellent device with which to activate the body by creating a variable resistance as well as a massaging effect.

13. For your endurance: Holding the towel by its ends across your back, inhale deeply. Now pull the towel forward, crossing your arms in front and exhale completely. Pull back, inhale. Repeat exercise.

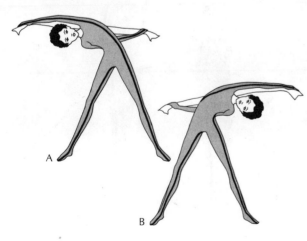

14. For your suppleness: With the towel stretched across the back of your neck, take a deep breath, circle your right arm behind your back, and bring your left arm up overhead as far as it will go, bending your body to the right. Exhale. Inhale while straightening up. Change arm positions and bend to the left, exhaling. Keep your arms as straight as possible.

15. For your equilibrium: Be sure you have enough room if loss of balance occurs. In standing position, hold the towel taut in front of you at waist level, hands apart the width of your shoulders. Try to pass your leg over the towel and back again. Repeat with the other leg. Exhale when your knee is highest and inhale when your leg is down.

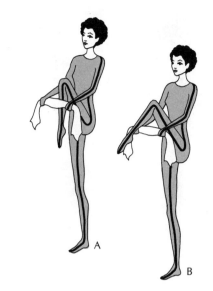

16. For your strength: Holding the towel taut behind your neck, one arm bent, slowly resisting, describe arcs from side to side, alternating arm bends. Inhale when arms are up, exhale when one arm is down. Graduate the intensity by increasing your resistance.

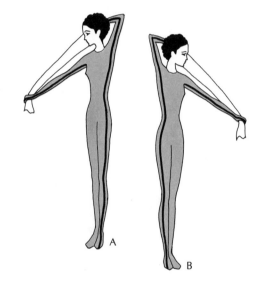

17. For your speed: In a solid lunge position, holding the towel in both hands, arms up and spread, body slightly arched, forcefully bring your arms down to the floor. Continue the exercise, accelerating the tempo, ten to fifteen times. Repeat on the other leg. Exhale, arms down; inhale, arms up.

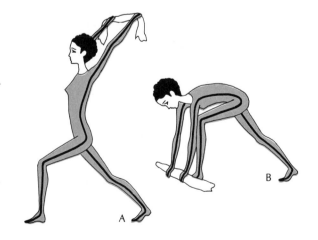

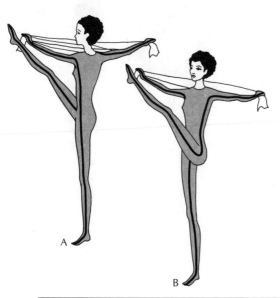

18. For your coordination: Standing upright, arms outstretched and holding the towel behind you, raise your right leg, twisting your trunk to the right, and try to reach your foot with your left hand. Alternate, inhaling when you are in a straight position, exhaling at the end of the twist.

INSTANT FITNESS WITH A BROOM

Use a broomstick as an aid for posture, as a support, or as leverage for twist. In order not to knock into the walls or furniture, you need space for these exercises.

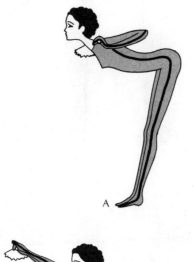

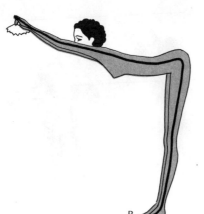

19. For your endurance: From a standing position, body bent forward, arms bent, hands holding the broomstick across the back of your shoulders, slowly, without touching your head, extend your arms up and forward. Inhale when arms are extended and exhale when arms are bent.

20. For your suppleness: In a sitting position, legs wide apart, arms outstretched, broomstick across the back of your shoulders, twist your torso, try to reach your foot with the opposite hand. Exhale when you reach down, inhale when you straighten up.

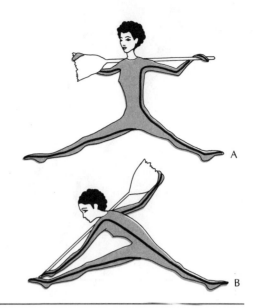

21. For your equilibrium: From a standing position, arms forward holding the broomstick and one leg extended behind you as far as it will go, move that leg forward and up several times, without losing your balance. Repeat with the other leg, inhaling when the leg goes down, exhaling when the leg goes up.

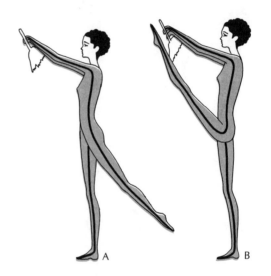

22. For your strength: Standing, legs wide apart, holding the broomstick vertically with both hands, its end resting on the floor in front of you, slowly bend one knee after the other, using the broomstick as support. Exhale bending down, inhale straightening up.

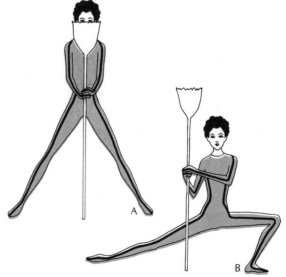

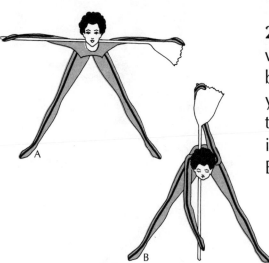

23. For your speed: Standing, legs wide apart, body bent forward, broomstick held across the back of your shoulders, proceed with caution to twist your torso, accelerating as you repeat the exercise. Breathe in rhythm to the exercise.

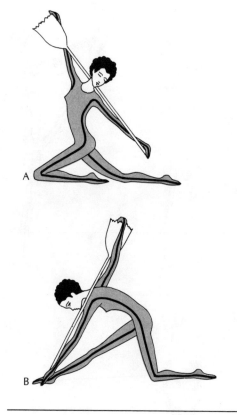

24. For your coordination: Kneel on your left knee, right leg extended behind you, broomstick held across the back of your shoulders, arms outstretched and torso turned to the left. Now, slowly twisting your body to the right, raise your hips and move your right leg sideways and forward, trying to reach the right foot with your left hand. Return to the original position and reverse the movement, kneeling on your right knee. Exhale when you are down, inhale when you are up.

INSTANT FITNESS ON A CHAIR

A straight chair is useful for several fitness exercises. Be sure the one you use is sturdy and stable.

25. For your endurance: From a sitting position on the chair, stand up several times in succession without the help of your arms. Inhale when up, exhale when down. This is good to keep the muscles of the thighs in shape, as well as to activate circulation.

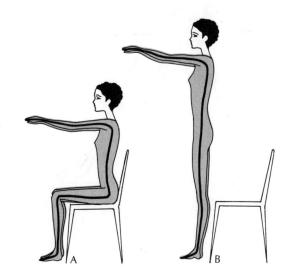

26. For your suppleness: Sitting on the chair, inhale deeply and bend forward to touch the floor, letting your breath out as you bend. Straighten up. Bringing one arm up and back, the other down and back, gently stretch your shoulders and spine as you inhale.

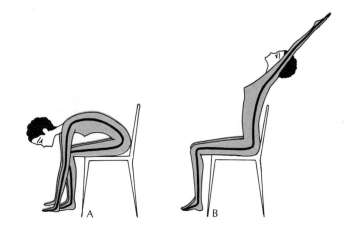

27. For your equilibrium: Sit on the chair, right hand holding the back of the chair, left hand holding the front edge of the seat, right knee bent, with the right foot on the seat, left foot on the floor. Releasing your arms, try to control your balance—first seated on the chair, then as you gradually try to raise your left foot and balance on the right. Breathe regularly, do not hold your breath. Maintain balance for about ten seconds. Now turn the chair or turn around and repeat on the other side.

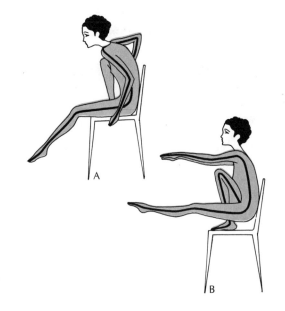

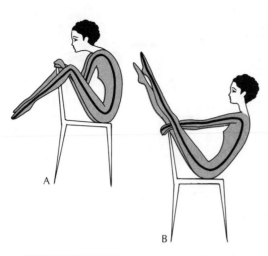

28. For your strength: In straddle position, facing the back of the chair, both hands on top of the back, raise both knees while bending forward and exhale. Slowly extending legs up, lean cautiously back and inhale.

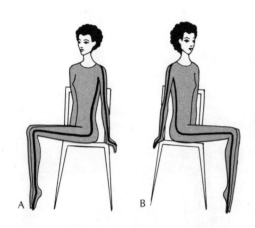

29. For your speed: Sitting deep in the chair and grasping the sides of the seat tightly, hold your legs together and swing them from side to side, accelerating the tempo, working up from ten to thirty times.

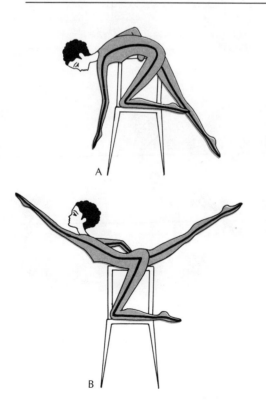

30. For your coordination: Kneeling on your left knee sideways across the chair, right hand on the back of the chair, left arm dangling down, raise your right leg and left arm, arch your back and inhale. Exhale as you return to your original position. Repeat several times, then turn around, change position and do the same, kneeling on the other knee.

INSTANT FITNESS IN AN ARMCHAIR

31. For your endurance: Sitting in the armchair with your shoes off, breathe deeply, bend your knees and hug them, rounding your spine. Exhale. Then open up, bringing your feet down and elbows back, and gently arch your spine, inhaling.

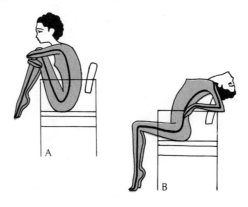

32. For your suppleness: Sitting on the edge of the armchair, bend forward, trying to reach your toes. Exhale. Then, supporting your body with your hands on the arms of the chair, and bending your right knee, lift it up as far as it will go, raising your hips and arching your body as you inhale. Repeat, alternating knees.

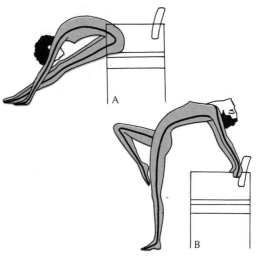

33. For your equilibrium: Standing behind the armchair, body bent forward, hands on the arms of the chair, find your balance point and carefully raise one leg and then the other and, if possible, both, gently arching your body. If assured of the position, try to balance with both legs and one arm up and, if possible, both arms up. Exhale when bending, inhale when arching. Proceed with caution: be sure the armchair is well-balanced and solid enough to support you.

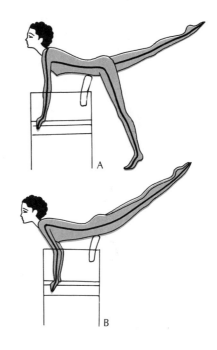

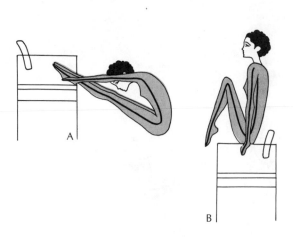

34. For your strength: Sitting, preferably on a carpet, legs straight, feet on the seat of the armchair, try to reach up and touch your toes with your finger-tips. Also, try sitting in the arm-chair, hands on the arms of the chair, bend and lift your knees, trying to push yourself up with your arms. Exhale when you bend, inhale when you relax.

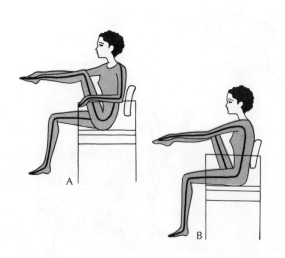

35. For your speed: Sitting in the armchair, as rapidly as possible bend one knee and touch your foot with the opposite hand, alternating sides and accelerating the pace. Breathe regularly at a slow tempo.

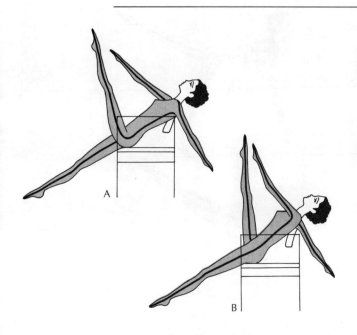

36. For your coordination: Sitting on the edge of the armchair, body straight, arms hanging over the sides of the chair, simultaneously and slowly try to raise one leg and reach the foot with the opposite hand. Alternate, exhaling when you touch, inhaling while you change.

INSTANT FITNESS AT THE DESK

Sometimes we spend several hours straight at the desk, without moving. The result is that the circulation becomes sluggish and all the muscles suffer from insufficient activity. Therefore, it's a good idea every hour or so to interrupt the immobility by doing some exercises.

37. For your endurance: Sitting at knees' length from the desk, hands clasped behind the head, move your elbows forward until they rest on the edge of the desk, exhaling as you bend. Then straighten up and, moving your elbows back as far as they will go, inhale.

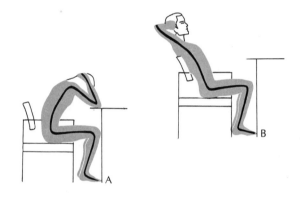

38. For your suppleness: Sitting at the desk, one hand on the back of the chair, the other on the desk, twist your body, exhaling at the end of each twist. Change arms, inhaling as you change and twist to the other side.

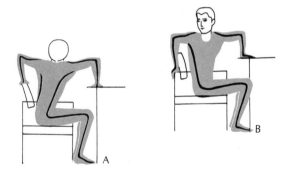

39. For your equilibrium: Sitting on the edge of your chair, arms outstretched, try to keep your balance while raising your legs and bending your knees one after the other. Breathe slowly and regularly.

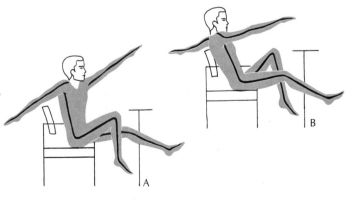

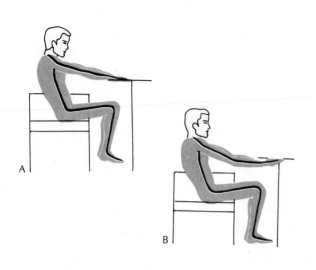

40. For your strength: Sitting with both hands on the desk, palms down, hands apart, apply pressure and hold it for a few seconds, varying the position of your hands from close to wide apart. Then place your hands, palms upward, under the desk, apply pressure and, again, hold it for a few seconds. Breathe deeply.

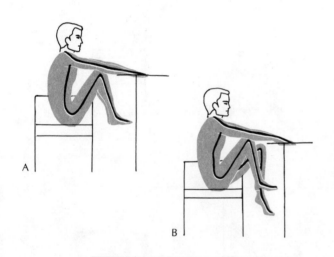

41. For your speed: With your chair a little away from the desk to make room for your legs, place your hands on the desk and try to imitate running and jumping motions with your feet. Do these motions for fifteen seconds each, accelerating the pace. Breathe normally.

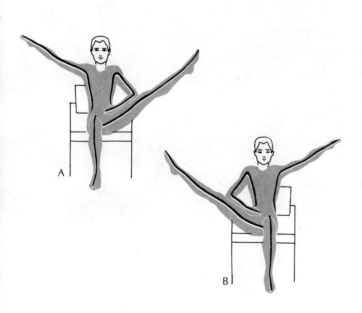

42. For your coordination: Sitting at the desk, your right arm outstretched to the right and your left leg extended to the left, your left arm bent, hand on hip, simultaneously reverse positions of arms and legs. Inhale as you stretch and exhale as you change positions.

INSTANT FITNESS IN A DOORWAY

Use your doorway as an instant gym. If necessary, make notations on the frame to mark your progress.

43. For your endurance: Standing across the doorway, both hands holding one side of the frame, raise your left knee and bend the other leg as far as you can without forcing, and exhale. Straighten your right leg and extend your left leg behind you, and inhale. Repeat several times. Then do the same gymnak with the other leg.

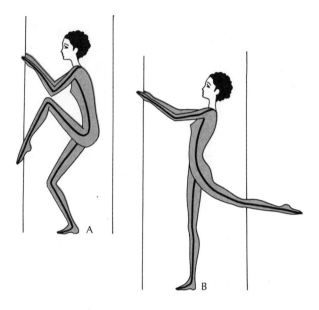

44. For your suppleness: Stand in front of the doorway with your back to it at an adequate distance (start close and move further away from it as you progress), arms up, hands holding the right and left doorframes. Now lunge back with your right leg, gently arching your body and breathing in as you go. Then lift your right leg forward and up as far as it will go, exhaling. Repeat a few times and then do the same with the other leg.

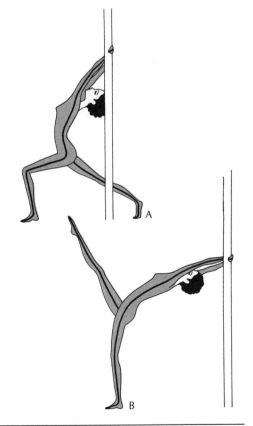

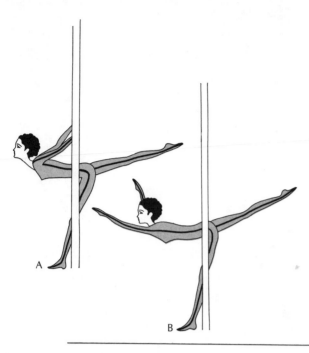

45. For your equilibrium: Standing in the middle of the doorway, both arms outspread to help your balance, extend one leg at right angles behind you and lean forward, trying to perfect your balance without holding the doorframe. Breathe normally. Repeat with the other leg.

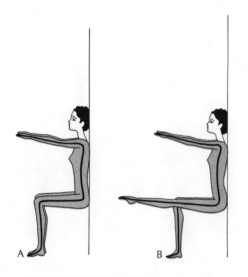

46. For your strength: Standing across the doorway, back against one side of the frame, place your feet at different distances and try to bend your knees, holding the position. Now try to straighten one leg. Breathe slowly.

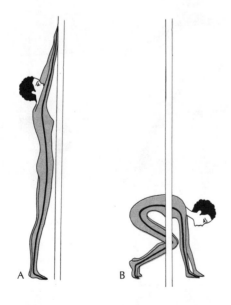

47. For your speed: Standing facing the doorway, try to touch the top of the door, then the floor. Repeat for ten seconds, trying to make as many bends and stretches as possible. Exhale when down, inhale when up.

48. For your coordination: Stand in the center of the doorway, your back to it, arms up and placed on either side of the frame. In a continuous motion, raise your right leg to the left and up, and your left arm to the right and down. Keep alternating. Exhale when the arm and leg are crossed, inhale as you assume your original position.

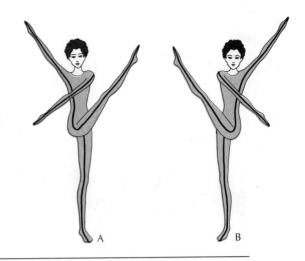

INSTANT FITNESS (STANDING)

No equipment or gadgets are needed here—just enough room for you to stand.

49. For your endurance: From a standing position, arms up as high as they will go, inhale. Lunge forward on one foot, bending your body and touching the floor with your hands, if possible. Exhale. Alternate legs.

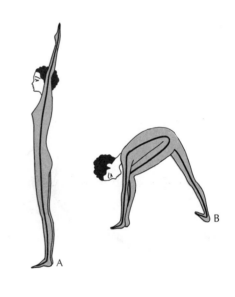

50. For your suppleness: From a standing position, take a deep breath, raise your left knee high, bend your body forward, moving your arms back and up, and exhale. Circling your arms down-forward-up, gently arching your back, move your bent knee back and up and inhale. Repeat with the other leg.

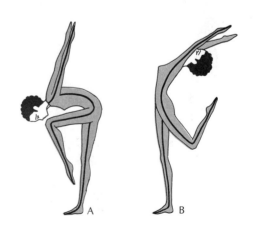

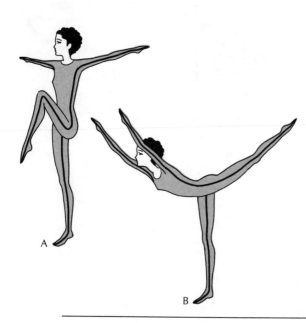

51. For your equilibrium: In a standing position, arms outstretched, left knee bent and raised, eyes closed, try to extend your left leg back and lean forward, balancing for ten seconds. Breathe regularly and repeat with the other leg.

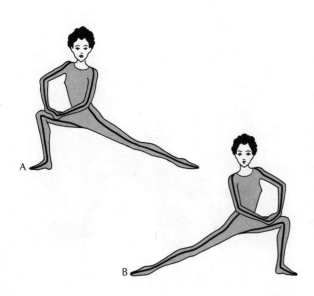

52. For your strength: Standing, feet wide apart, turning your body to the right, bend your right knee as deep as possible and exhale. If necessary for balance, you may use your hands placed on your bending knee. Straighten up, inhale, turn to the left, bend your left knee and exhale.

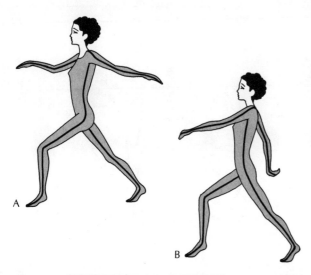

53. For your speed: Standing on your toes in a half-lunge position, swinging your arms, imitate running in place, rapidly changing the position of your arms and legs. Breathe as needed, with as slow a rhythm as possible.

54. For your coordination: In a standing position, raise your left arm up, extend your right arm and left leg sideways and inhale. Bend your left knee in and up and exhale. Slowly move your right arm forward, your left arm back, gently arching your back and inhale. Repeat with the other leg.

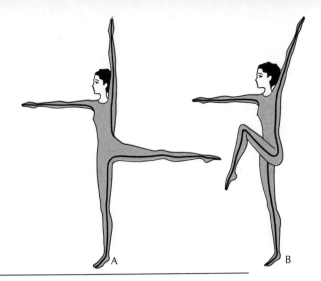

INSTANT FITNESS (PRONE—SUPPORT)

For efficient work or pleasure, for tasks or games, the entire front of your body must be fit.

55. For your endurance: From frontal support on hands and feet, leaning carefully on your arms, lift your hips and gradually spring forward and back, approaching your arms. Breathe rhythmically and deeply. Exhale when bent, inhale when extended.

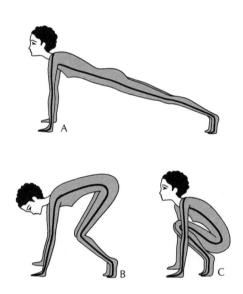

56. For your suppleness: In a kneeling position, knees and body bent forward in front flexion, arms straight forward and down, exhale. Slowly, keeping your knees bent, rise up on your hips and inhale. Now lower your body forward, arch your back and using one arm for support, bring the other forward and overhead as far back as possible. Repeat with the other arm.

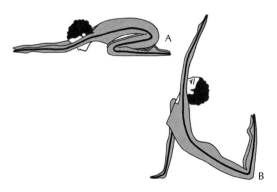

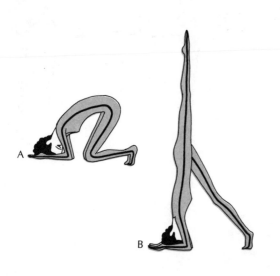

57. For your equilibrium: From a kneeling position, bend forward, elbows at right angles to your body, palms up with one hand over the other, and place the top of the head on your palms. Leaning on your elbows, hands and feet, slowly raise your hips, straightening your legs, and extend one leg up, getting used to the upside-down position. Return slowly to the kneeling position. Repeat with the other leg. Inhale when leg is extended, exhale when it is bent.

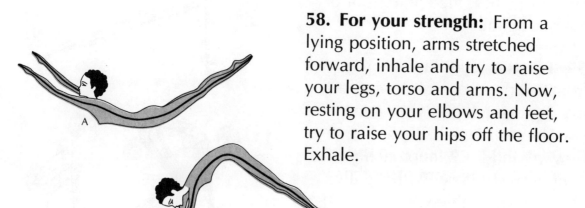

58. For your strength: From a lying position, arms stretched forward, inhale and try to raise your legs, torso and arms. Now, resting on your elbows and feet, try to raise your hips off the floor. Exhale.

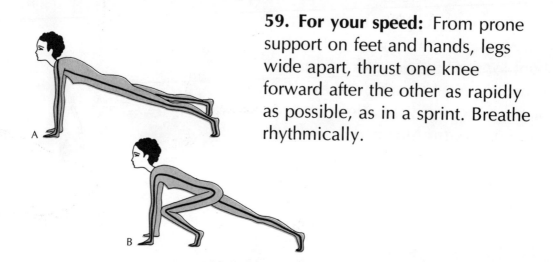

59. For your speed: From prone support on feet and hands, legs wide apart, thrust one knee forward after the other as rapidly as possible, as in a sprint. Breathe rhythmically.

60. For your coordination: In prone position, elbows bent and pulled back, legs up and bent at the knees, slowly extend your left arm and right leg. Alternate, extending the opposite arm and leg. Breathe regularly.

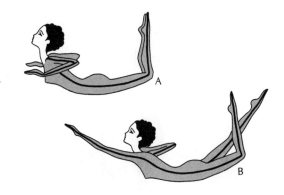

INSTANT FITNESS (LYING—DORSAL SUPPORT)

There are certain actions, such as sitting down on the floor and getting up, that now and then you may be called upon to do—with grace, we hope. To be able to do these takes fitness.

The following gymnaks may take a while to do properly. In the beginning use your arms or other support if needed. If you find the whole exercise too difficult, do only the first gymnak in the set, working up to the second or third as your skill improves.

61. For your endurance: From a standing position, arms forward, slowly bend your knees, lean forward and sit down, exhaling. Now lie flat and bring your legs up over your head. Swinging your arms, torso and legs forward, and bending your knees, try to stand up, inhaling as you rise.

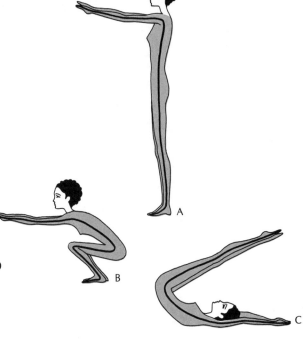

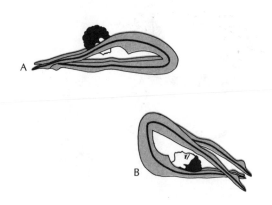

62. For your suppleness: From a sitting position, body bent forward, arms stretched trying to reach your toes, exhale. Inhaling, swing back, rolling on your spine and spreading your legs. Try to reach with your feet as far back as possible, using your arms and upper back as support. Exhale.

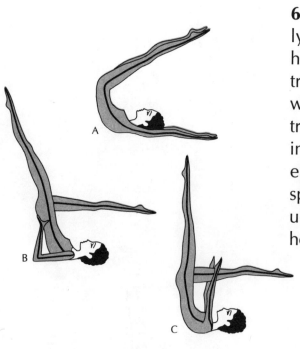

63. For your equilibrium: From a lying position, arms stretched overhead, lift your legs and hips and try to balance on your upper back with the help of your arms. Then, try without using your arms. Placing your hands on your hips with elbows as support, slowly try to split your legs forward and back, ultimately balancing without the help of your arms. Breathe slowly.

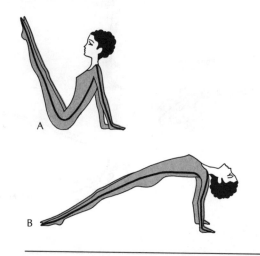

64. For your strength: From a sitting position, arms back, leaning on your hands, raise your legs and exhale. Lower your feet and, raising your hips, arch your back and inhale. Now, lower your hips and assume your original position. Repeat.

65. For your speed: Supporting your body on your arms and the soles of your feet, one knee bent, bounce gently, changing legs, and accelerating the pace as you go along. Breathe according to your needs. Five to ten times each leg.

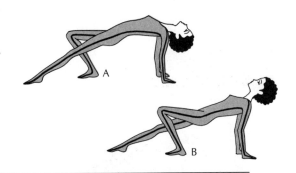

66. For your coordination: From a sitting position on the floor, left knee bent, left arm extended behind you for support, raise your right leg as high as possible and circling with your right arm, pivot to the left and try to stand up on your arms and left leg. Repeat with the other side. Inhale sitting, exhale turning.

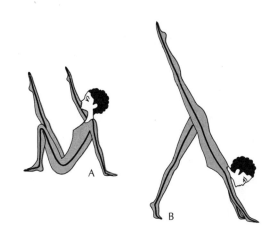

INSTANT FITNESS IN THE CAR

Exercising in the car is a safety measure, and it also gives you a chance to catch up on your six minutes of gymnaks a day.

On a long drive, pull off the road, stop the car and try these gymnaks to reduce fatigue and tension.

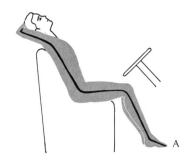

67. For your endurance: Sitting comfortably, hands clasped behind your head, move elbows forward and in, rounding upper back and neck, exhaling. Open your elbows out, arching your upper back and neck, inhaling.

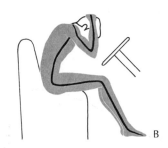

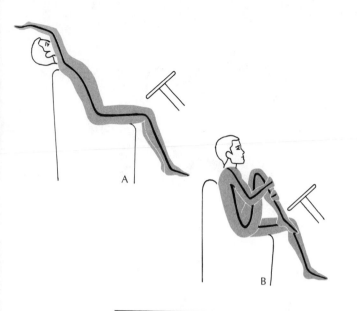

68. For your suppleness: Sitting deep in the seat, linking your fingers, raise your arms and pull them overhead, inhaling. Now carefully bend one knee, hug it, and pull it as close as you can toward your shoulder, exhaling. Repeat with other leg.

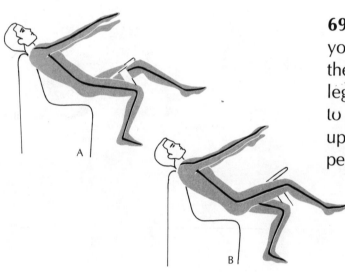

69. For your equilibrium: Pressing your shoulders against the back of the seat, one knee bent, the other leg straight, raise your hips and try to balance on one foot and your upper back. Breathe normally. Repeat with the other leg.

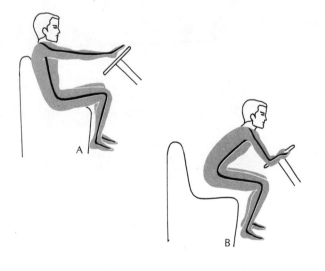

70. For your strength: Sitting deep in the seat, hands pressing against the steering wheel, contract your abdomen, pressing your back against the seat and exhale. Now, with the help of your arms, holding the steering wheel, try to lift your hips off the seat, inhaling.

71. For your speed: Let the car seat back as far as it will go. Sitting firm, feet apart, hands on chest with elbows at shoulder level, twist your body from side to side at a gradually accelerated pace. Breathe steadily.

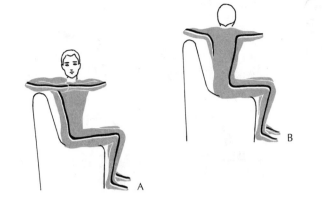

72. For your coordination: From a sitting position, feet apart, fingers clasped behind your head, twist your torso and raise one knee, trying to reach the knee with the opposite elbow. Repeat on alternate sides. Exhale when you twist, inhale in straight position.

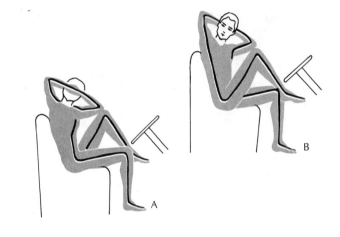

INSTANT FITNESS OUTSIDE THE CAR

73. For your endurance: Supporting yourself with your hands on any sturdy part of the car, make a series of knee bends from light to deep. Start gently, exhaling when down, inhaling when up.

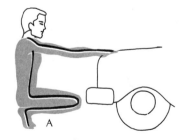

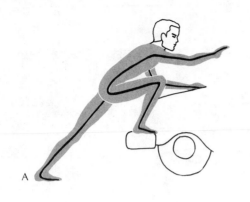

74. For your suppleness: Place one foot on a protruding surface of the car, such as the bumper, and lunge deeply, alternating legs and supporting yourself with one hand. Exhale as you lunge, inhale as you change legs.

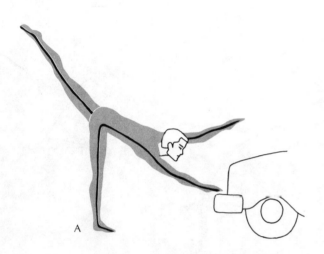

75. For your equilibrium: One leg up, body bent forward as low as possible, try to keep your balance for about ten seconds without touching the car with your hands. Have your arms ready to restore your balance, if necessary. Breathe deeply. Repeat with the other leg.

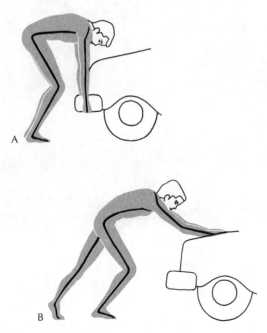

76. For your strength: Place your hands under the car at the bumper, feet placed comfortably. Make an effort as if you were lifting the car. Then place your hands on the car and from a comfortable stance make believe you are pushing the car. Exhale as you make the effort, inhale as you relax.

77. For your speed: Standing, feet together, hands on the car, try to spring rapidly, raising your hips, bouncing into the air with your feet apart, landing with your feet together. Breathe rhythmically.

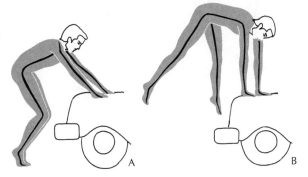

78. For your coordination: From a standing position, lunging forward on one leg, extend the opposite arm up and forward. Return to your original position, change leg and arm, and repeat. Exhale when lunging, inhale when upright.

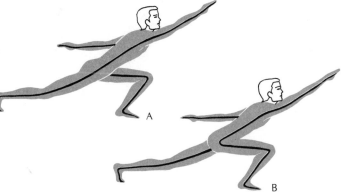

INSTANT FITNESS FOR SUPERSTARS—WOMEN

Once you are in top form and can call yourself a superstar—and if you want to remain one—it is important to do some demanding exercises regularly. These gymnaks are certainly not for the beginner and are probably too exacting even for the intermediate student.

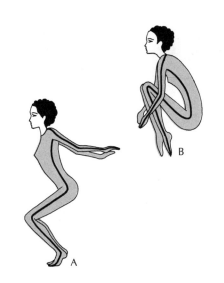

79. For your endurance: At a continuous pace on your toes, try to spring up in the air, simultaneously bending your knees and hugging them as in a kangaroo jump. Breathe rhythmically.

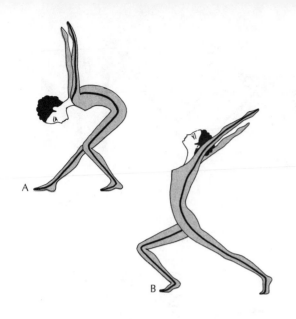

80. For your suppleness: Right leg forward, left leg back, flexing the left knee, bend your body forward as you circle your arms back and up, and exhale. Reverse the circling direction of your arms, extend the left leg behind you and, bending your right knee, shift your weight forward in a lunge position, raising your arms and arching your back as you inhale.

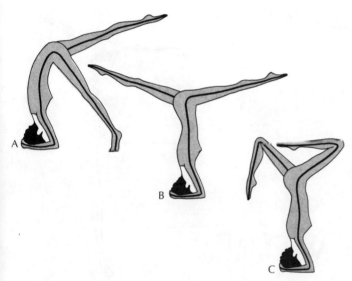

81. For your equilibrium: Forearms on the floor, palms up, one over the other, the top of your head inside your hands, legs straight, hips up, slowly raise one leg until you reach the split position. Controlling your balance, simultaneously bend both knees, then, straightening your legs, return to the initial position. Breathe deeply, slowly and rhythmically.

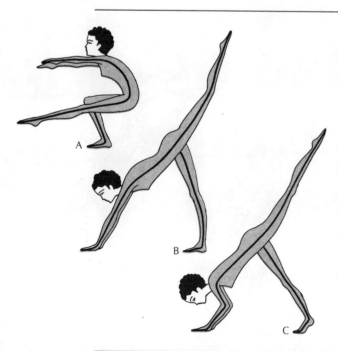

82. For your strength: From a sitting position on the floor, the knee of one leg bent and, pressing with that leg, slowly lift yourself up, moving the straight leg back and up. Then, placing your hands on the floor, return to the initial position. (For men: the exercise should be completed in a deep push-up.) Repeat with the other leg. Exhale sitting, inhale reaching up.

83. For your speed: From a support position on hands and feet, half bend one knee, keeping the foot on the floor. Springing and bouncing, change the position of the legs as fast as possible, breathing rhythmically.

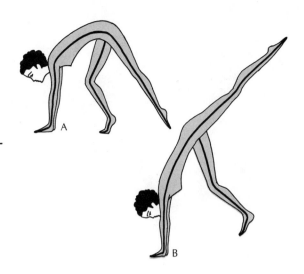

84. For your coordination: Balance on your left leg, body bent forward, right arm down, right leg outstretched sideways to the right, left arm outstretched to the left. Slowly straightening your body, move your right leg forward and up, your right arm up and your left arm forward. Repeat with the other leg. Exhale while bending; inhale straightening up.

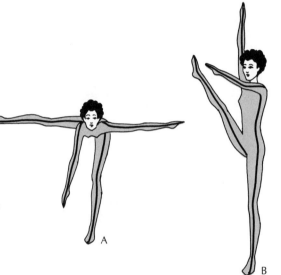

INSTANT FITNESS FOR SUPERSTARS—MEN

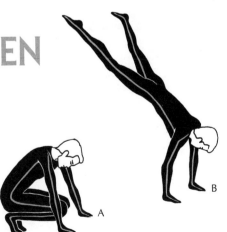

85. For your endurance: With your knees bent and supporting your body with your hands on the floor, in a continuous springy motion bounce your legs into the air, your legs wide apart. Breathe rhythmically.

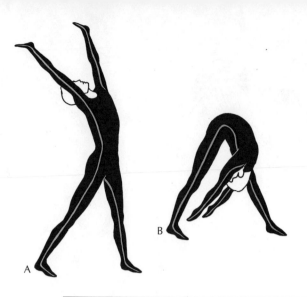

86. For your suppleness: Standing legs wide apart, bend your body forward, swinging your arms down and back as far as you can reach and exhale. Then, straightening your body, arch your back and inhale.

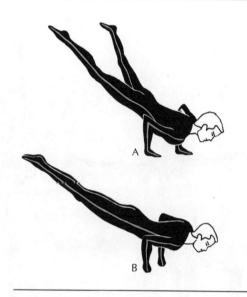

87. For your equilibrium: In a prone support position, hands and feet on the floor, arms bent, legs wide apart, fit your right elbow in under your hipbone and try to find your balance. Then raise your feet off the floor. Repeat with other arm, breathing steadily.

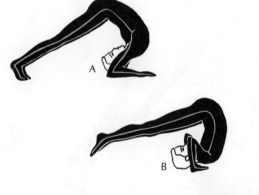

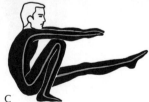

88. For your strength: Body bent forward, hands and feet on the floor, curl your head between your shoulders and bending your arms, rotate forward in a somersault, bending one knee and coming up on that leg to a standing position. Repeat on the other leg. Exhale as you bend, inhale as you stand up.

89. For your speed: Bounce fast to a split position, changing the position of your legs with each bounce. Breathe rhythmically.

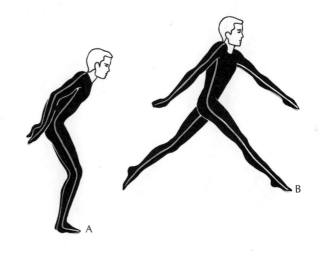

90. For your coordination: Balance laterally on your left leg, body bent to the left, right leg and left arm in stretched horizontal position, left arm down. In a sweeping lateral motion change legs, leaning to the other side. Exhale as you lean down, inhale as you come up.

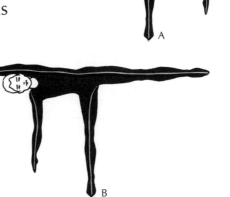

12

TO FITNESS WITH LOVE

Once understood and properly pursued, fitness becomes a friend who will help us live well and enjoy every minute, heightening our senses and brightening our spirits.

Unless we devote a few minutes a day to fitness, the downhill path to "unfitness" can be followed in no time at all. Then fatigue and its consequences—irritability, tension, stress and exhaustion—will slowly sabotage our health and happiness.

The best way to avoid unfitness is to have a preventive program that we follow regularly to recharge our batteries, tune up all systems, eliminate poisons and toxins, eradicate bad habits and improve our bodily assets—in short, to stay fit.

Fitness gives us spiritual, mental and physical balance. It makes us healthy, it makes us look and feel good. As a plant gets a little water or sunshine and then straightens up and blooms, or a bird in the fresh air spreads its wings and flies freely, proper exercise gives an astonishing lift to body and spirit. It gives us that great feeling of elation and satisfaction with ourselves and with the world that can only be described as happiness.

So—to fitness, with understanding and appreciation!

About the Author: Nicholas Kounovsky, the author of several exercise books, including *The Joy of Feeling Fit,* is perhaps the world's leading exercise specialist. He has appeared on numerous radio and TV shows, and more than two hundred articles on him have appeared in leading magazines and newspapers in the United States and around the world. Mr. Kounovsky, trained in Europe and the United States, lives on Long Island and is an enthusiastic tennis, volleyball and paddle-ball player.

His credentials include:

Honorary Diplomate of the Ministry of French National Education;
Graduate of the Sokol Method of Gymnastics in France;
Licensed automobile and aeronautic construction engineer;
Graduate of the Swedish Institute in New York;
Chief Instructor of the American-Russian Sokol;
and former director of the Nicholas Kounovsky Studio in New York.